101 Positive Affirmations for Women : A Workbook

101 Positive Affirmations for Women : A Workbook

Award-Winning Author Dr. C. Topjian

Authors Get Published

Authors Get Published

Contents

101 Positive Affirmations for Women

A Woman's Wellness Curriculum Guide & Workbook

By Dr. Christine Topjian

101 Positive Affirmations for Women

Published by Christine Topjian Publishing
(An Imprint of Authors Get Published)
www.AuthorsGetPublished.com
www.DrChristineTopjian.com
Toronto, ON

Introduction

You've heard it before and it is so important that it is worth repeating: speaking positively over our lives is so important, so vital, so necessary and wisdom says it is worth our time to engage in the practice each and every day.

Our self-talk is part of the building blocks of how our lives will shape up to be. Speaking to ourselves and over ourselves with positive, life-affirming, Christ-centered words, sentences and phrases is necessary and should be an everyday practice. Not only does the world respond to what we say to ourselves and out loud, but our subconscious mind is also listening, hearing, absorbing and much more. You are either creating and producing more life, or you are destroying it. Which will you select?

What are you telling yourself each day? Are your messages positive and life and goodness affirming? Or do you talk down to yourself, telling yourself you are no good, have no value and that you do not have worth.

Take it from me: you have worth. You are wonderful and worthy and you are deeply loved by Jesus. I don't even know you but I don't have to know you to make that statement. Jesus is perfect and if He chose to die for you, then He knows well enough to put His stamp of approval on you and to tell you that you are awesome. We are all works in progress because we are not perfect but a work in progress is still valuable.

This book is specifically for women and it is your invitation to be good to yourself, to love yourself and to treat yourself with much love and kindness. The words and the affirmations included in these pages are specifically designed for women of all ages, sizes, colors, backgrounds, etc.

This book is a workbook specifically dedicated to you and designed for you, the empowered woman, and to help you make it a daily, habitual process of helping yourself to look, feel and be your best.

Please take the time to do the exercises, to answer the study questions with all honesty and to say the affirmations either out loud or in your mind. Repeat them over and over again. You will get the most out of this book if you go through all the exercises and you dedicate a bit of time each day or so to complete the exercises. We all have busy lives (I get it) but we all need to make time for our growth, our wellness and to invite Jesus' power into our lives.

Shall we get started?

A Bit About Why This Book Was Created

It was a crisp summer evening and we were going to have family over for an occasion. Among the guests was one lady who walked into the event speaking so negatively about herself and speaking as though she did not recognize her own value.

I noticed this and found this to be worrisome. I began asking myself "How many women out there are speaking negatively over their lives and saying negative, disempowering, self-defeating things about themselves?" "How many are doing this without even realizing it?" As I began to listen more carefully to diverse women around me, women in church, women talking to their friends at coffee dates, women in the workplace, I began to notice that many do. Many women do not speak well over themselves and have gotten into the unfortunate habit of doing that. They say words like "I'm no good at this", "I'm just not very smart", "I'll never get anywhere in life" and much more.

That's when inspiration for this book happened.

It is meant to be a guidebook and to serve as a consistent reminder to each woman out there that we need to speak well over ourselves and that this needs to be a regular practice. As humans, it takes time to learn things, to fully adopt new ways and to change the way we speak and the way we think. I also saw this as an opportunity to provide examples of the positive words that we need to speak because many out there are not sure what to say to themselves. They are not sure which words to speak that will help empower them and improve their lives. So, I believe a manual was needed to help women all over the world learn to speak properly over their lives and to help bring good things into their lives, through the goodness and powers afforded to us through Christ's sacrifice for us.

Just a bit of back information for those who may not be fully aware: When Christ died on the cross at Calvary, He did it as a sacrifice so that every single person who believes in Him will have the opportunity to tap into that goodness because all power has been granted to Him, so when we believe in Him and we pray in His name, we are evoking the benefits of that sacrifice. Each and every time we pray in His name. Why would we not partake in that benefit each day?

I pray that this workbook will be your go-to resource for this. I pray that this will be a guidebook and a reminder to start and to continue doing the exercises, to continue writing your responses and to use the empowering words provided in this workbook and if you would like to add some of your own, that's fantastic! You can use the space provided at the back of this workbook to write them out. Feel free to take this workbook with you as you go about your day, as you go out with friends and family, to refer to during your prayer times, when you are looking after your kids, etc. There is no end to the amount of positive action you can take to bless your own life.

A final word about the reflection questions included at the end of each chapter that you will be asked to respond to: please do these and answer them to the best of your ability because they will help you get a better sense of where you are and where you want to go. Remember to pray through these questions and to be honest with yourself.

This entire workbook is meant to be a journey you take in tandem and in partnership with the Lord, who loves you beyond what you can imagine and fathom, and who will speak to you via the Holy Spirit. Ask Him to * journey with you * ask Him to show you things you may not have realized * ask Him to guide your responses and answers for best results * ask Him to give you visions of what is good and best for you * ask Him to help you through each step of the process.

Remember also, we are not here to be perfect. We are here to be the best possible versions of ourselves in Christ and by leaning on Christ.

Happy reading and experiencing!

Appendix: The Wisdom in Repetition

There is great wisdom in repeating something worthwhile over and over. It is with repetition that we, as humans, really get something down. It is by repeating it over and over again that we really learn something and that it gets down into our most precious subconscious. When it gets down into our subconscious, we begin to act with more gusto, we begin to take on more empowering decisions and choices and we begin to really work strategically for our best lives.

Some women may feel awkward about doing that. I get that but powering through that and really taking the strategic actions of repeating these positive affirmations again and again will be tremendously beneficial to your life.

Enjoy yourself with this workbook. Say your empowering words out loud or to yourself as many times as you like. Say it in different ways, in different intonations, and with different mannerisms. Use an accent to make it more fun if that works for you. Enjoy this process! And if you are doing these activities with a group, feel free to show them your zaniness and your unique and fun personality. People love to see that in others and respect when someone demonstrates their unique talents and abilities while working on becoming a stronger woman.

Life in Christ was always meant to be enjoyed!

I Love Me

Living a more empowered and more positive life starts with you loving yourself. It starts with you cherishing yourself and with you realizing that you have great value. Just as you are.

Of course it's important to want to improve ourselves and to better ourselves mentally, physically, emotionally, etc. But we need to realize that we deserve to be good to ourselves today and now, and that we do not suddenly become worthy of love when we've lost weight or when we start to style our hair a certain way or when we finally land this job or that one. Now. Here. Today. You are awesome.

Loving yourself means being good to yours and therefore, the world around you will treat you the way you project yourself to be treated. If people are not treating you the best right now, it may be a bit of a reflection on how you have been viewing and treating yourself. If that is you, consider this your official invitation to change that and to lead a life where you command more respect. Commanding more respect is in your hands and when you begin to be more positive and make more positive statements, you will begin to see things changing and shifting on the outside as well. For some, this may be a novel concept (and that's ok)...the point is to begin and then, to keep it up.

For example, people can sometimes be disrespectful. They could be having a bad day, they could be annoyed, or they could just not see the value in treating someone well all the time. If we allow them to be disrespectful to us and to speak to us in ways that are rude, demeaning and unkind, then we are letting them know that they are allowed to mistreat us, that we allow them to be unkind to us and ultimately, that signals to them that we do not respect ourselves enough to command their respect.

When you get into the practice of standing up for yourself in a manner that is gentle but firm, you are creating a context for yourself to be treated well by others. You are elevating your own worth in your own eyes and in the eyes of others. This is very important because ultimately, how we allow others to treat us is a reflection of how we treat ourselves and how we communicate to them how they are supposed to treat us. If you see your own value, you will insist on people treating you very well and this will promote people being good to you because you have set that benchmark. Conversely, if you don't see your own value, you will not make it a point to command being treated well and you will not insist on that being part of your daily life.

Never underestimate the power of one single interaction. One person who treats you as less than.

Sometimes, people can write off how someone treats them one time. Don't. Every interaction is important and during every interaction, the person needs to treat you with utmost respect. If they don't, the incumbency is upon you to gently but firmly communicate to them how you expect to be treated and addressed. Never underestimate the power of one single interaction. One person who treats you as less than.

I remember one woman I had met recently (as of this book's writing) who used a term when referring to me that I really didn't appreciate. I found the term a bit demeaning and not at all appropriate. I gently but firmly mentioned to her that I didn't like the term and that I didn't want to be called that term, especially since the term did not in any way apply to me. I let her know that I didn't like it and why and that I am sure she did not mean to be disrespectful but that I found being called that word disrespectful. She has never done it since and I set my boundary for a more respectful relationship.

This applies to career, family, relationships, friends, etc. When you see your own value, it demonstrates to others that this is a woman that demands (rightfully so) to be respected, to be treated right.

Wouldn't you like that? Wouldn't you like and enjoy being treated with respect always? That is not something that just happens - it is a benchmark we must set for ourselves.

So, it is the way you speak. It is the way you carry yourself. It is the way you dress. It is everything about you.

To provide an example, I was recently looking at pictures of a beautiful Hollywood starlet online. She was exceptionally beautiful, very wealthy and seemed to have so much going for her. And then I began to notice the way she carried herself. She did not carry herself in a classy way. In the photos, she was with the man she had just married and she carried herself in a way that showed that she did not value herself. She carried herself in a way that did not indicate that she commanded any respect for herself. She had posted photos of herself looking less than classy and in a way that did not reflect that she commanded respect.

Now, I am not saying that you cannot or should not be fun-loving and have lots of great energy and enjoy life. Of course you should! But there is a very big difference between classiness and having a fun time versus being less than classy and not holding yourself up to the best possible light.

How we show ourselves matters. How we carry ourselves in public matters. How we carry ourselves indicates to others that this is a woman who values herself, who respects herself and with whom I need to be respectful. People learn that they have to treat you with the same respect that you command for yourself.

In the same way, how you speak over your day, your week, your month and your life matters. Saying negative and derogatory words like "I'm an idiot", "I'm no good", "I'll never get this right," "I'm worthless", and such are not appropriate, kind or constructive ways to speak about yourself. Carrying yourself with your shoulders slumped or with your appearance not properly groomed are not the best ways to carry yourself. It is our right and our duty as women to value ourselves and to respect ourselves by carrying ourselves well and by treating ourselves with the same respect with which we expect others to provide us.

If you feel the world is not respecting you in the way that you would like, please look critically for a moment at how you treat yourself. Do you demonstrate a respect for your own self? Do you speak well of yourself? Do you speak and act in a manner that commands respect for yourself?

I witnessed a situation some time ago at work. A woman was being confronted about something her boss wished she had handled differently. He was speaking to her very respectfully and I believe his choice of words was appropriate. In return, she raised her voice significantly, let him know that she was not happy with his perceived evaluation of things and began yelling expletives at him. I can understand frustration in the workplace (I think it's fair to say that we have all been there) but what isn't acceptable and isn't commanding respect and love for oneself is raising one's voice and reacting the way that she did. We can choose better.

Speak Positivity!

There are many ways (and variety of words) anyone can use to speak positively about yourself and over yourself. It is not overdoing it to speak positively several times each day, reminding yourself of your worth, how wonderful you are and that you are a gift of God. Now, I want to be clear that building yourself up and speaking well over yourself is very different from being stuck up or self-centered. At some point, most women can feel down about themselves, for one reason or another. It is fairly normal for us each to have days or moments when we don't feel good about ourselves. The trick then is to pull yourself out of it and to remind yourself of your innate awesomeness, your wonderful qualities, your fantastic gifts and the fact that you are a work in progress. I will explain that last point just a bit more: none of us is perfect. We are all works in progress and that's ok. We all have to take on the conscious role of accepting that we are not perfect but that we are working at being better each day. This workbook's intent is to be a tool to help you remember, practice, think and speak your self-worth each day.

You are never alone in reminding yourself of your self-worth. Instead, you are in daily, even hourly partnership with God and He is the One who can help you and lift you up when you are not feeling your worth in those moments.

Prayer for Help

Prayer, as I always say, is our right and our privilege. Prayer is asking God to help us and to raise us up. It is our birthright and our way of communicating with God about anything.

As such, in those moments when you are not feeling your best, I'd like to offer this prayer so you can feel raised up:

Dear Lord, I'd like to ask You in this moment right now to help me remember my worth. I am asking You to help me feel like Your child because that is what I am. In my moments of feeling low, like right now, I ask You to raise me up, remind me of how wonderful You have made me, of my talents, my skills, my abilities, and why I am so wonderfully made. Please help me to remember that You, not the world, hold the keys to my worth and I ask You to build me up right now, Lord. Build me up, please, and remind me of my worth. In Jesus' mighty name.

Amen

Here are some ways to speak positively and in a way that is empowering. There will be a total of 101 in this workbook. Since this is your workbook, feel free to mark up the page by highlighting sentences and phrases that resonate with you and speak to you and feel free to make jot notes as you go. Feel free, also, to make amendments to the sentences provided here to make the affirmation work more readily for you. The affirmation has to resonate with you, ultimately.

1. I am beautiful, I am smart and I am worthy.

2. I am deserving of the very best.

3. I am kind to others and I deserve to receive kindness in return.

4. I love being good to myself and I respond well when others are also good and kind to me.

5. I respect myself and as such, I remind myself each day that I am deserving of the respect of others.

6. I love myself and as such, I remind myself each day that I am deserving of the love & respect of others.

7. I am an intelligent woman.

8. Good and valuable people love spending quality time with me.

9. I am worthy of all goodness, including love.

10. My mistakes do not define me.

11. I am a valuable woman. I am a valuable human being.

12. I work hard and I deserve praise and accolades at work.

13. I am there for my family and my friends and I deserve respect, kindness and caring from my family and friends.

14. I treat strangers kindly and with respect and I deserve and receive that same kindness and respect from strangers.

15. I am a beautiful, intelligent woman.

16. I am a person who is valued. If others do not see my value, I can move on from them.

We can never underestimate the value and impact of our words. Think about it....when you speak positively over yourself, you feel better. When you say something positive to someone or pay them a compliment, they feel better. It is scientifically proven that using good, kind and positive words help to lift depression, increase and improve self-esteem, helps to bring people joy and overall, is a win-win-win for anyone involved. We have enough negative things coming at us and negatively impacting our day - saying negative things about ourselves is not going to be what we need. But the fact is, people need regular reminders to be and to stay positive. They need reminders around their living spaces and even on their devices (like a smartphone) that remind them that they are good, valued, loved and more. Many people that I know choose to couple their daily affirmations with daily Scripture devotionals - that is also a fantastic idea!

Devoting Time to This Practice

Sometimes, we may think of engaging in these mental health supports and practices, but a distraction can come, a negative news report can happen or someone says something thoughtless or unkind and then we can simply forget the good. It is very easy for this to happen and it is very easy to slip back into the old habit of either not speaking positively or not reminding ourselves of our value. This is why I suggest keeping positive reminders and notes around you.

Grab a sticky, a piece of paper or your device. Better yet, grab all of them and write reminders for yourself to get into this practice and to be consistent at engaging in it. Make the reminders easy to access and readily present because when we are in the middle of a busy day, we need the reminders "there" and readily available to us. Even if we are not in a toxic or difficult situation in our personal or professional lives, not reminding ourselves of our value will begin to chip away little by little at our sense of self worth and then after a short time, we will see that not engaging in these uplifting practices has cost us more than we have initially realized.

New Phases

When you are entering a new phase in your life (no matter what that phase is or at what point in your life that is happening) and you are on a learning curve, doing this practice of reminders and affirmations is vitally important. Let me illustrate: when we are entering a new phase, such as being pregnant or starting a new job, we are inevitably going to be on a learning and experiencing curve. We are not going to get everything right the first time and we are going to make mistakes. When we aren't sure of what we're doing or we feel like we aren't being at our best, we can easily start to feel bad about ourselves. That's when we have to catch ourselves and remind ourselves that we are working at it, we are trying, we are doing our best and we are moving forward in the right ways, praying for God's guidance and protection as we move forward.

Questions

1. On a scale of 0-10 (0 being the worst, 10 being the best), how would you rate your current view of yourself?

2. Do you currently believe that you speak well over yourself and your life? Why or why not?

3. Do you feel or believe that you were ever taught (as a child or later in life) to speak well over yourself? If so, how do you feel about that? If not, how do you feel about that?

4. Do you want to learn to speak more positively over yourself and your life? Are you willing to commit to doing so?

5. Do you believe that this is in your power?

6. Are you willing to work at this each day? There is no problem with putting a reminder for yourself in your phone, notes or anywhere else that might be helpful for you so that you have a reminder to continue working on this each day. It is only by working on it each day and being consistent with it that we are going to see results. Jot down where you are going to put reminders for yourself and what reminders would be most helpful and empowering for you.

2

Why You Should Believe in You

All of us have goodness, and talents in us. Each and every one of us does, no matter where you are born, the color of your skin, whom your family is, what mistakes you have made, etc. We all have goodness in us and we deserve to have a good and happy life for ourselves, in tandem and in partnership with God.

This is one of the main reasons Jesus died for you and I on the cross at Calvary. That's right - He believed you and I and the next person are so special that He died to give us life, relationship with Father God and happiness.

You Are So Valuable

This is a really important point to continue making. You are so valuable. If you were told as a kid or at any point in your life that you were less than completely invaluable (that means immeasurably valuable), I'd like to tell you that that isn't true. You are valued, valuable, wonderful and amazing. Just as you are.

When people feel badly about themselves, they can (and do) take that out on others, especially when they know that promise, talents, skills and goodness resides within that person.

A man I knew was a wonderful, kind, encouraging soul. I do not believe he had one nasty bone in his body but all his life, he was told by his adopted mother that he was worthless, that he was a waste of space and that he would never amount to anything. She even told him (at the age of about 13) that she regretted adopting him. That will destroy a person inside. She had no right to destroy his sense of self and to make him feel like nothing. He grew up to be a wonderful adult, kind and respectful of others and employed in a profession where he works to make children feel better, learn, and grow in a space that is safe, caring and loving. He strives to give others the loving space that he never had. Talk about turning a negative into a positive!

It's A Reflection Of Them, Not Of You

When people speak negatively over you or about you, know that it is because they don't feel good about themselves. It has nothing to do with you. So when someone says or implies negative things about you, the best thing to do is to move away from that person or persons as much as you can because they are trying to poison your world instead of improving their own.

Here are positive things you can say over yourself if you were (or are) in that position:

17. I am a valuable human being. If others see that in me, then that's great but if they don't, it doesn't take away from my goodness.
18. I am beautiful, smart and well-equipped for every good work Christ guides me to undertake.

19. The right people enjoy being with me and spending time with me.

20. God has equipped me for every good work.

21. God has wonderful plans for me.

22. I am physically, mentally, and emotionally a masterpiece. God put His awesomeness into me.

23. God created me on purpose, to bring joy, goodness and happiness into the world. The world is better off because I am in it.

24. The Lord has wonderful plans for my life and I intend to see those plans through.

25. No matter what negatives others may have said about me in the past, I am a wonderful, valuable woman.

26. God created me as a wonderful, blessed, joyful woman and I love being me.

The Beauty of You

God knew very well what He was doing when He created you. From the time you were being formed by God in your mother's tummy, He created you to be a wonderful, intelligent lady and an asset to the world. I don't need to know you personally to know how true what I just said is. I know that God is perfect and does not make mistakes, therefore, I also know that He only creates wonderful works and masterpieces - so I know that you are one of His masterpieces.

We just need to make sure that you see yourself accordingly.

27. My beautiful _____(insert the color of your hair) hair is lovely and I style it beautifully.

28. My _____ (choose one or more body parts) is or are beautiful and beautifully-formed.

29. My hands, feet, nose and mouth are an artistic work of God and so they are beautiful, at the exact size that they are.

30. I am the perfect height for me. I am neither too tall nor too short. Just perfect.

Questions

1. On a scale of 0-10 with 0 being the lowest and 10 being the highest), how do you currently rate all of the following attributes of yours:

   My physical features: _____

   My mental wellness: _____

   My emotional wellness: _____

   My intellectual capacity: _____

2. Name at least five things you love about yourself. Please be as detailed as you would like.

   a)

   b)

   c)

   d)

   e)

3. When you pray about improvements, what do you feel the Holy Spirit is saying to you about what is already wonderful about you?:

4. If you are a woman who grew up with disempowering words, phrases and more thrown at you consistently, and you now recognize how damaging those words were, are you willing to make a conscious decision to set aside those disempowering words and opinions of another and instead, take on good and empowering words and opinions? Are you willing to realize and accept that those mean, terrible and nasty words were nothing more than an attempt to make you feel bad and to bring you down by someone who feels horribly about themselves? Write out your thoughts and reflections about that here. If you need more space, you are free to use the space in the back of this book. I have left additional space there for this very purpose.

If you don't feel that you have a relationship with the Holy Spirit and find it difficult or challenging to invite the Spirit to help you answer these questions, here is a suggested prayer you can use to assist with this:

Holy Spirit, I thank You for loving me and for residing within me. I would like Your infinite knowledge, help and goodness to help me through this part of my process for improvements. I am asking You to come into my heart in an active way and to show me what I need to see in terms of improvements. I am asking You to show me what I need to do in order to get better. Please speak to my heart clearly and tell me what is needed and what steps will be needed for improvements. In Jesus' name. Amen

3

Your Wonderful Physical Attributes

So often in our day, we see images of seemingly-perfect bodies, and seemingly-perfect lives. These images do affect us and while we have made progress in terms of having more realistic body figures represented in the media, we can still easily get down on ourselves. We can feel like we are overweight, undesirable and not attractive or not attractive enough.

We need to remind ourselves each and every day (sometimes more than once a day) to really focus on helping ourselves feel better and building ourselves up with strong, empowering words, sentences and phrases of affirmation.

It is so important to help ourselves in this way because feeling good each day should be the norm. I know that for some women reading this, it may seem like a daunting task to remind yourself of your worth and your physical beauty each day (next chapter deals with mental beauty) but we have to start today (this very hour, really) in order to make this a regular, daily habit. We have to make our health an everyday practice - a go-to practice where we tell ourselves that we love exactly how we are and who we are, just as we are. Of course, we should be working each day on improving ourselves with such things as eating well, going to the gym, doing our yoga and our workouts and much more. These are things that will help us feel better and operate better in our day.

I always like to say regarding workouts, the mentality shouldn't be that we have to work out, but that we get to work out.

I always like to say regarding workouts: we get to work out. We get to walk, run, sprint, and do weights. We get to be good to our bodies by exercising and eating well. We get to do body-enhancing activities and mental-health boosting things because ultimately, we will benefit big time from these actions. We get to do these!

31. I am great at working out and I enjoy it.

32. I work out and do body and mind-enhancing activities every day.

33. I choose workouts that work for me and that safely push myself to greater levels and greater heights.

34. I am a working out work in progress.

35. I am making great progress in my workout process.

36. My health is improving every day.

37. I find new workouts that are great for me and that push me to greater accomplishments.

38. My workouts and my yoga and breathing practices are like a love-letter to my body, my mind, my spirit and my soul.

39. I dedicate myself to working out _____ minutes per day.

Whether you do a small workout or a little one, the point is you are making that time for wellness for you. And the benefits of this permeate through all parts of your body and all parts of your mind. I always feel so refreshed and wonderful after doing a workout, especially when it involves cardio and really pushing myself safely but surely. I know that we all have busy days but making the time or setting aside the time for this will benefit you and all those you come into contact with.

Eating Well

Again, so important: we need to eat well-balanced and nutrition-filled foods such as proteins, vegetables and fruit, whole grains and legumes. When we eat well, we are fueling our bodies for the day and we are giving our bodies the vitamins and nutrients it needs to be healthy and to keep going.

Personally, I believe that all the nutrients we need come from the foods that we eat, as long as we are selecting healthy options. I don't take supplements for that reason and don't really feel that I need them very often. Of course, if your physician has told you that you are in need of certain vitamins, go right ahead if you want but generally, if we are eating very well, all the vitamins we need come from well-selected foods.

Toxic People

There are toxic people all around us. I define toxic people as those who are regularly negative, speak negatively and are not positive or optimistic in any way. I also include in that list people who may not speak or say negative things around you or about you but don't have good or positive vibes toward you. Listen, of course we all have bad days where we want to vent, to air out our frustrations or to just talk something out - but it becomes a problem when we are doing this regularly and causing ourselves and others to feel so sapped of energy. This is an actual phenomena - we can sometimes get ourselves so down that we get sapped of energy - you can literally feel the energy being sapped from your body.

We must surround ourselves with positive, optimistic people and we must practice being so ourselves.

The people we surround ourselves with are going to have a tremendous impact on us, whether we like it or not. People who are negative will be (one way or another) causing us to be more negative and the reverse is true too. We have to remember that we are susceptible to the influences of others and we have to ensure that we are building ourselves up with our own words, our own prayers, with Christ's goodness and protection and with the people we choose to have around us.

Here are some reflection questions for you for this chapter. Remember to answer as honestly as possible - this is meant to be a helpful tool for you to bring to light any issues, thoughts and things that are holding you back from living your best life.

1. On a scale of 0 - 10 with 0 being the weakest (most negative) and 10 being the strongest (most positive), how would you rate your own level of positivity? How do you feel about the rating you have given yourself?

2. On a scale of 0 - 10 with 0 being the weakest (most negative) and 10 being the strongest (most positive), how would you rate the level of positivity of the 5 people who are closest to you? Name each of the 5 people and put the rating scale of your choice next to their name. How do you feel about this rating?

3. On a scale of 0 - 10 with 0 being the weakest (most negative) and 10 being the strongest (most positive), how would you rate your level of positivity from 3 years ago? The purpose of this question is to gauge and reflect on whether you have become more positive or more negative in the last few years.

4. On a scale of 0 - 10 with 0 being the weakest (most negative) and 10 being the strongest (most positive), how would you rate the level of positivity of your parents or guardians? This is an important question because we often emulate what our parents and guardians say and do. We were raised by them and so we have to factor in that their example has had a significant impact on us and has influenced our own outlook.

5. How many days per week do you currently engage in at least 15 minutes of physical activity? Are you happy with this number?

6. Are you willing to dedicate yourself and commit to increasing your level of physical activity? Using a percentage scale, and if you said yes to dedicating yourself to an increase, how committed will you be to this increase (ex. I am 100% committed. I am 50% committed. I am 75% committed.)? If you did not say yes to being dedicated to an increase, I suggest you reflect on why you are not willing to be dedicated and perhaps you can partake in our supportive message boards at www.drchristinetopjian.com to get some support from others who have also created a profile and have chosen to engage in our support forums.

7. How willing are you to dedicate yourself and commit to increasing the amount of positive speaking you do daily? Using a percentage scale, how committed will you be to this increase (ex. 10% dedicated, 80% dedicated, etc.)?

8. Write down 3 positive affirmations you create (you can use any of the ones provided in this chapter as a reference or a starting-off point) and practice saying them out-loud or in your mind. Feel free to take your time with this. These are your affirmations and they are meant to improve the quality of your day.

I really want to emphasize in closing this chapter the importance of dedicating yourself to speaking positively over your physical life. This is so important because each day we get is a gift to do great things and to accomplish great things. Tomorrow is not promised. As such, focus on the good and bring more of it into your life. You do benefit tremendously from doing this and so do the people around you.

One last word I'd like to add regarding women with physical

disabilities: you are beautiful and lovely. Whether you feel ok or not about your physical disability, I would like to note that your physical disability does not make you any less lovely and beautiful. You are still awesome and lovely and you are still meant to and invited to do life with God. I have great respect for people who have disabilities of any kind and who choose to do their best and to work their hardest, despite any challenges.

4

Your Wonderful Mental Attributes

Our mental health is simply vital. We have to protect our mental health and when we take Jesus out of that equation, we are battling in vain because it is Jesus that is going to help us improve in leaps and bounds. It is through His sacrifice on the cross that we are afforded the ability to defeat any and all evil thoughts that come and that try to bring us down. By taking Jesus out of the equation, we are literally battling on our own and in vain.

We Are Sheep

For those who may not be familiar with Biblical teachings, God refers to us as sheep. Sheep are precious animals but they are vulnerable and so they need their shepherd (God) to help them, to keep them safe, to protect them and more. It is really important to remember that when we take God out of our lives and out of the equation, we are on our own and that we are fighting battles on our own. Praying for God's protection and bringing Him into the equation is essential because we are then able to access His help, His protection and His goodness.

Our mental health needs to be protected each and every day, not just once in a while. We have to remind ourselves of our worth, of the beauty that is within us and of how great we are. God chose to create you just as you are and He does not make mistakes.

The world around us will seek to bring us down. We can have colleagues, family and friends who may feel jealous or envious or just not wish the best for us and therefore will try to bring us down. Knowing this, we have to work on our own self-concept by remembering who we are in Christ and to protect our mental health. We have to cover ourselves with the blood and protections afforded to us by Jesus in order to engage in effectively protecting ourselves, helping ourselves, advancing in life with His power behind us and to feeling good each day.

Activities That Help Us Feel Good

Whether it is taking a nice long walk, having a fresh cup of water, buying ourselves flowers, listening to uplifting music, taking a drive in your car or in your vehicle, giving yourself a tap on the shoulder, or simply writing "I love me" in your journal, activities and actions such as these are vital to our daily positive mental health, to our self-esteem and to our wellness - and we need to engage in these activities each day, sometimes a few times per day.

If you don't yet know what activities would help you feel good, or you have an idea but you aren't yet sure, may I suggest starting one or two or three and see how you feel doing each? These activities are meant to enhance your happiness and if you have never thought of doing things like this before or you have but you haven't engaged in anything like it yet, this too may feel like a daunting step. Relax. It is meant to be enjoyable and you are meant to have fun with it. Slowly, you will begin to identify what makes you feel good, what makes you happy and what makes you feel calm. And if something works for someone else but doesn't for you, not to worry. You will find what works for you. Sometimes, it is simply a matter of making a few adjustments and you can easily adapt something to suit you and your needs. Simply put, just because something works for one person, it doesn't mean it will also work for you. Be gentle with yourself and slowly see yourself going through the task, seeing if it works for you and maybe, with small tweaks as you are going, it will be for you.

To illustrate this, I'll take the example of two ladies I know well, Maddie and Jane. Both find great comfort and solace in taking leisure walks in their respective neighborhoods. Maddie loves being among trees, grass and greenery while Jane loves the feeling of walking slowly because she and her late dad used to take long walks together and that was her way of connecting with him. Maddie loves to go quickly on her walks and that provides her with great enjoyment and mental health peace, while Jane hates walking quickly and finds that more stress-inducing. When Maddie saw that Jane was doing this activity to feel good, she took this very advice and started to make tweaks to her lifestyle so that she could do these walks as well. Same activity, done more than one way, works for two different women in two different ways. Beautiful!

Dedicating Yourself

When I suggest dedicating yourself to figuring out which activities would be good for you, I mean it and I say this respectfully: *we are all busy but we have to find the time to do these good things for ourselves.* If we do not, we are not helping ourselves and regardless of what your home or work situation is, you owe it to yourself to find the time in your day (yes, once per day at least) to do something meaningful for you.

So, the question begs: Are you willing to dedicate at least a bit of time each day to doing something meaningful for yourself and your mental health?

I hope you answered yes to that because when we don't take care of ourselves, dear ladies, we will feel the effects, we will not be at our best and we will risk making things worse for ourselves.

The Breath

Here is an important point I'd like to make for those days or those moments when it is particularly hard to find a moment to yourself or when you are feeling overwhelmed: take a breath. Breathing is so so important and is so cleansing for our minds, bodies and souls. If you can manage to get outside for a few minutes to take a few nice deep breaths, then that's great but even if you can't get outside or get to a window, taking those deep breaths inside can also do wonders for you.

Breathing helps us calm our bodies and our minds. It helps us gain some perspective. It helps us feel more in-tune with ourselves and you regain that feeling of "Ok, I am getting my head on straight again." Don't cheat yourself of that time.

40. I breath deeply each day and it helps to calm me down.
41. I dedicate at least 20 minutes per day to doing activities that are good for me.
42. I am great at taking some time for myself even in the midst of a busy day.
43. I rely on God to protect me and to keep me safe.
44. I am grateful for all the love and the protection God provides me with.

Questions:

1. Name some activities that help you feel good about you. Use the space provided here to do so. There are no limits to the number of activities you put down so if you need to continue on the spare pages provided at the back of this book, please do so.

2. Ask yourself for a moment: how many deep, cleansing breaths do I take in a day? This is not the same as regular automatic breathing. No. This breath I am referring to here denotes purposeful, deep, expressive breath where you hold the clean air in after breathing in very deeply and holding it in for a moment before you let it back out. If you are not doing this a few times per day, I'd like to suggest you mindfully take some more time in your day to do this.

3. How much water do you drink in your day? Drinking water

is extremely important for our bodies and we need to be drinking throughout our day. Some people don't love or look for water but we need to consume it. May I suggest you keep a running count of your water intake as you go through your day and however much you do currently drink, consider adding another glass.

5

Your Wonderful Intellectual Attributes

You are a lovely, beautiful woman. You are intelligent, you have so much good in you and you have gifts and talents that are meant to be shared with the world.

Are you honoring your own intellectual attributes?

45. I am an intelligent woman.
46. I am smart.
47. I have many interesting and important things to say.
48. People love to hear me speak and they learn a lot from me.
49. I read quality materials that the Holy Spirit guides me to and I regularly pick up new ideas and new concepts.
50. People enjoy talking to me and they really, deeply listen to what I have to say.
51. I respect my own mind and my own abilities.
52. Positive thoughts flow from me regularly.
53. The Lord has given me a beautiful mind and beautiful abilities.
54. I regularly think good and positive thoughts about myself.
55. I regularly think good and positive thoughts about others.

56. People seek me out for my thoughts and input and then implement them.

57. My intellectual input is valued at work.

58. My intellectual input is valued at home.

59. My friends, colleagues and family all love to ask me for my thoughts and opinions.

60. I am a kind, generous person.

61. I laugh at least once a day because it is good and cleansing.

62. God has created me with a sound mind.

Saying Your Affirmations

At this point in the book, I'd like to take a moment to remind you to say your affirmations, stick up post-its and notes with these messages for yourself around the home, put these reminders in your phone and your devices, and really take the time to make it clear to yourself that you are saying these words to yourself and that they are meaningful. Even if it is a bit hard to believe positive things about yourself today, when you make this part of your lifestyle, it will become natural and if you open yourself to it, it will begin to positively affect your life.

Many women I know who have gotten into the wonderful habit of doing this have taken to saying it to themselves in the mirror. They enjoy seeing themselves say these words in the mirror and they enjoy how they feel afterward.

Please do so as well if that works for you. When you take the time to implement and actually do the exercises taught in this book, you will not only get so much more out of this book but you will also have gotten into the habit of engaging in this important practice for yourself.

Remember that what you put into it, you will get out of it. There are no shortcuts to this.

In Privacy

Many women will prefer and will choose to say their affirmations in private. And that's ok. If you have to go to your car or to the bathroom or anywhere you feel is private enough so you can comfortably say your affirmations, please do so. Do these affirmations in a way and in a space that feels the best to you because the main thing is you are doing them in a self-loving and positive way. It would not make sense for you to say your affirmations in a destructive way.

Questions:

1. How much time do you spend each morning or day reminding yourself of your intellectual worth?

2. How much time do you spend each day reading and gaining new knowledge? Are you willing to increase that a little bit?

3. Are you willing to look in the mirror and say your positive

affirmations about yourself? Why or why not? If you said that you are willing to, I'd like to congratulate you. If you said that you are not willing to, I'd like to invite you to pray about that decision and ask the Lord to show you the benefits of an exercise like this.

4. When you have tried the affirmations for a week, I'd like to ask you to write down how you are now feeling about yourself. Are you feeling any better? Do you sense small but important changes in yourself? Describe those for yourself in as much detail as possible. Remember that you can come back to this exercise and to your responses (I would date them if I were you) so you can see just how far you have come in progress when you look back on this later on.

6

Your Powerful Inner Circle

Your inner circle is one of the most important things in your life.

You tend to listen to your inner circle. You tend to trust your inner circle. You tend to go to them for input and for advice and you rely on each other. Your inner circle is important to you and rightly so. I would like to encourage you to make sure that the members of your inner circle are cherishing you and honoring you the way that you deserve to be cherished and honored and that when you select your inner circle, you consult with the Holy Spirit on who should be included.

My friend Myla did not have that luck at first. Her inner circle was one that she fell into by default and unfortunately, they were not being good or kind to her. One was always jokingly putting her down, the other was not really there to help her but instead, acted quite selfishly, while the other was unfortunately floundering in her own life so she was not a very positive influence. Myla felt sad all the time because she was looking for validation from her inner circle but there was none to be found. She had always dreamed of a great inner circle and while she hadn't yet found it, I advised her to pray about it and to ask God to bring her the right circle. I can tell you that many changes took place for her that year and she now has a very thriving inner circle.

Please make sure that you have prayed about whom you allow into your inner circle and when you have gotten that information, that you are connecting with them, learning from one another, and building each other up in good and constructive ways.

63. My friends love me and cherish me.

64. My friends and inner circle treat me wonderfully.

65. My friends and inner circle respect me deeply and show me that respect on a regular basis.

66. I have a wonderful, God-given inner circle.

67. My inner circle spends time each day or week building each other up, supporting each other, and pushing each other to strive for better, more, and higher.

68. My inner circle and I pray together.

69. My inner circle and I have formed a prayer chain and pray for each other regularly and in emergencies.

70. My inner circle is one given to me by God.

71. The loyalty we have to one another is astounding and I am very grateful for it.

72. My inner circle and I trust each other.

73. We always have each others' backs.

74. When I feel angry or frustrated with my inner circle, I pray for God to give me His wisdom and His perspective on how to handle it.

75. My inner circle and I give each other time and space when we need it but we always still really know how to be there and support each other.

76. My inner circle and I always speak uplifting and kind words to each other.

77. We attend church and Bible studies together.

78. I am so grateful for my wonderful inner circle.

If you already have a wonderful, life-affirming inner circle that the Holy Spirit has guided you to, that's wonderful. If you do not, pray for the Lord to bring you that. He will do so and you will slowly see things shift in that direction and for the right people and circumstances to present themselves to you. Always pray over new happenings to verify that they are from the Lord and in an effort to not be deceived. He may ask you to go somewhere new. He may ask you to do something different. He may ask you to gain a bit of distance from this person or from that one. If He does that, know that He knows best and He is leading you away from something that He knows will not be the best for you.

Many people are of the understanding that just because something happened or materialized, that that is from God. Not so. The enemy can also make things happen. So we need to pray and discern with the Holy Spirit so that we do not get in the practice of relying on our own wisdom.

I will never forget when the Lord guided me away from a friend I had had for a long time. It felt really hard at the time because I felt that she and I were quite close and I really didn't want to believe that she could have anything but the best and most noble of intentions. Unfortunately, His guidance to move away was really quite clear. As I began to move away from her, I began to really think about and reflect on her past words, past actions and the way she had guided me over the years or suggested things I should do. I began to really see that her actions and her words were not all that loving. It was a very hard reality to face and I too, of course, also looked at what I could have done to have contributed to a less-than-stellar friendship. The more I thought about it, the more I realized that this lady was no longer meant for a friendship with me and that the Lord was (of course) correct in His evaluation. It was a hard and sobering realization to come to but that I really needed to be mindful of and stick to.

My suggestion to you is to pray over those you choose to have in your inner circle and then pay attention to how the Lord is guiding you. He may be guiding you toward one person or more and He may be guiding you away from another. He knows best and He knows you best.

Questions:

1. Write down the names of those in your current inner circle. There is no limit to the number of names you can put down. Be honest about this.

2. Pray over the names you have put down. What do you believe God is telling you about each of the people you have put down? Write down any thoughts, feelings and sensations you feel you are getting about this.

3. Ask yourself if you fully trust each of the members of your inner

circle. Trusting each person deeply is so very important. That trust is not to be taken lightly. They are blessed to have you in their lives and to have you trusting them so fully. Ask the Lord what He wants to say to you about this too. Ask the Holy Spirit to be very clear with you on this and to really reveal all that you need to know and to see about this.

7

Don't Give The Critics An Opportunity

Simply put, I believe we all have critics.

Criticizing someone with negative or less-than-positive intent is something critics enjoy doing. Critics are not there to be nice or constructive in their criticism. Constructive criticism exists to help you realize areas where you need to improve and are meant to make you better. Critics are not there to be constructive or to help you to improve. They are there to make you feel bad, and to tear you down.

It is up to you if you will open yourself to those opportunities. I don't suggest you give them those opportunities because being faced with their criticisms will only make you feel worse. *People can say what they want but it is within our control how we respond and if we will respond.*

You don't need to listen to any critics and you shouldn't. We are all human and as such, we all make mistakes. We all fumble and we all say and do things that we shouldn't. Critics are there to make you feel as bad as they can with negative intent. That is why you should stay as far away from them as you can and if you cannot stay away from them physically, it is in your power not to pay any attention to them.

I remember very clearly some critics that I have had in my life. They were people who tried to make me feel stupid, worthless, and like I couldn't do anything right. One person even laughed right in my face when I expressed legitimate concern about the mental health of a child I was teaching and who had just experienced a breakdown. That was one of the saddest professional moments because that wasn't at all about me, we were talking about the well-being of a child.

I am sure you have also had critics in your life and can recall how badly they made you feel. If we dwell on their criticisms, we are letting them get the better of us. That is not what we need to do. We need to hold our heads up high and keep moving forward, become or keep being positive, doing what is best, doing what we know is right. God sees the injustices and it is His place to vindicate you.

I'd like to suggest you feel free to move away both mentally and physically from those critics and to go on and build and live your best life. Take comfort in knowing that people who try to tear you down do so because they are trying to make themselves feel better. It's a cheap tactic on their part and you don't need to pay any mind to them. You have important things to do in your day and in your life. Focusing on them and their garbage isn't one of them.

Focus on your positive affirmations instead. Where your attention goes, your good vibes will flow.

79. I believe in my abilities.
80. I am a fantastic and wonderful person.
81. I may have some critics but I do know how to silence them: by paying no mind to them.
82. I am a happy person who is living her best life.

83. I am a work in progress and I am improving and getting better each and every day.

84. I am grateful for the errors I have made and the corrections I have made / am making because they are leading me to be a better person.

85. Jesus thought I am to die for and He is never wrong.

86. I can do all things through Christ who gives me strength.

87. The challenges have come but I don't have to get stuck on them.

88. I choose where I will focus my thoughts.

89. I decide what I pay attention to.

90. I have critics but I am choosing to move away from them today and every day.

91. I am a beautiful, vibrant, confident woman.

92. I spend time with Christ each day, affirming my incalculable value in Him.

Pray For The Strength

Praying for strength when the going gets tough is really important. It is really important to make that time and to really reach out to Christ, asking Him to give you all of the following:

- Strength
- Wisdom
- Perspective
- Direction
- Focus
- Remind you who you are in Him
- Ask Him to show you how to deal with the situation
- Ask Him to help you know your worth in the face of naysayers
- Ask Him to highlight Bible passages in your mind you can read that highlight just how valuable you are

- Ask Him to highlight Bible in your mind that remind you of just how to hold steady in the face of challenges

I remember I was going through a really tough challenge a few years ago. I had people around me who were making me doubt a new professional direction I knew God was leading me to take and I knew that I had to make a decision: I was either going to listen to Him or I was going to listen to those people. I took a long time to make the decision but ultimately, what got me through it was praying through it and asking Him to illuminate my mind about the truth behind the criticism. After much reflection, it dawned on me that those people had told me to cease the new venture because they wouldn't have been able to undertake the venture and they were trying to project that onto me. I was almost dumbfounded by the realization and I could see that I could easily take on this new venture and that I needed to dedicate myself to it in spite of some people around me saying otherwise.

Listen carefully and always trust what God tells you in any situation. He knows what He has put in you and when you stop listening to Him and start listening to others, that's when you begin to make your mistakes.

Questions:

1. When you think of your critics, are you willing to ignore them and to move forward positively?

2. Pray about what God would say to you about each of the critics you are thinking of in your mind. See what He wants to say to you about each. There may be things about them that you are not realizing.

3. Are you staying strong in who you are in Christ despite the critics? Reflect on what helps you stay strong.

8

Why This Book Doesn't Tout "Self Help"

> Life was always meant to be lived in partnership and in tandem with God and so if you feel alone, know that God is there to help you, to love you, to guide you, and to make you realize just how much He wants to bless you.

Simply put: we were never meant to do this life alone.

Life was always meant to be lived in partnership and in tandem with God and so if you feel alone, know that God is there to help you, to love you, to guide you, and to make you realize just how much He wants to bless you.

Self-help generally means doing it alone and having "the universe" bring something to you. It means relying on your own self, your own resources, and your own abilities for everything. I instead like to say that we are to rely on our work in partnership with God. We are not to rely only on ourselves. In the Bible, it says that we are sheep (and that's not an insult). Sheep are beautiful animals and they need their Shepherd to stay safe and to keep out of the wolf's way. If we are not staying near to the Shepherd, we are going to risk getting into some serious trouble, just like in the example of the sheep.

No matter who you are, where you are, what you've done or what you will do, Jesus loves you so much and He is asking you to rely on Him for all of the following:

- Your family life
- Your work life
- Your well-being
- Your future
- Your marriage
- Your mental health
- Your physical health
- Any and everything you need to do and will need to do

Some people don't know that God cares about us so much - even the little things. He wants you to come to Him with all your problems, questions, concerns, wonderments, insecurities, and the list goes on.

I remember watching an episode of one of my favorite tv shows and in it, a husband and wife were arguing about what they should pray for. The woman wanted to pray for something that seemed trivial (a new pair of luxury shoes to be very much discounted) and the husband was telling her that she was wrong to pray for such a thing. "God's a pretty smart guy...I think He can handle it" she countered. Well, she was right. God is very smart and nothing is outside of His reach and His abilities. She was not only right in praying for something trivial as well as the important stuff but she did end up getting those luxury shoes at a serious discount!

God does not care if it is 2 am or 2 pm. He is God therefore He neither sleeps nor slumbers. He is there, He is ready and He is available, waiting for you to go to Him and ready to be the Lord of your heart.

Please do not think you have to do life on your own. When He leads you and guides you, it is in a direction that He knows is best for your life, even though you may not be seeing that yet and He will provide all the help, guidance, open pathways, resources and more.

93. I lean on Christ for all my needs.

94. Christ gives me the strength I need to take on each day.

95. The Lord's strength renews each morning.

96. I am so loved by the most powerful God. All is under His authority.

97. Jesus loves me. This I know.

98. My power and my strength is found in Christ and will never expire.

99. I am a strong woman because Christ lives inside of me.

100. The doors that I need opened will be opened by God, in His ways and in His timing.

101. I love me and Christ loves me.

Questions:

1. Are you telling yourself and reminding yourself about Christ's love for you each day?

2. Are you telling yourself that you love you each day?

3. Are you believing in Christ's love for you and that He will be there to support you through anything you are going through?

4. Are you spending quiet time along with God each day?

5. Have you thanked Him lately for His blessings upon your life?

6. Have you thanked Him for bringing this book into your hands, meant to increase your self-love and your reliance on Him?

Reader, it is no coincidence that you picked up this book. Whether you got it from the bookstore, the library, a friend or a family member gave it to you, it is in your hands because God loves you and He wants you to know just how much. He wants you to rely on Him and He wants you to know that He is there for you through absolutely everything and anything. So lean on Him today and speak your words of life. They will do a great deal for you and they will help you realize your worth and your value.

He wants you to rely on Him and He wants you to know that He is there for you through absolutely everything and anything.

If You Are Not Sure How To Advance

If you are someone reading this and you are not yet sure how to advance and how to have God be an important, central figure in your life, I invite you to read on. I will provide a prayer you can pray where you invite Him and you can slowly start to see His power in your life. You can slowly start to see just how important and beneficial it is to have Him in your life.

Jesus,
I don't know You well but I am willing to come to You
And to ask You for Your help.
I am asking You right now to reveal Yourself to me and to show me what I need to do, how I need to do it and how to be in relationship with You.
I need You to go slowly but surely and I need You to reveal Yourself to me in any ways that You are willing.

You know my heart and You know my soul. Reveal Yourself to me slowly and show me how I can begin my own personal, loving relationship with You.

Thank You. In Jesus' name.

Amen

Here is to your best!

My Prayer For You With This Book

This book was written with the intention to help each and every female out there. If this book is in your hand and you are reading, I am grateful for that. I would like for this book to help as many women as possible, so if you can think of a friend, family member, colleague, etc., who would benefit from this book and its positive messages of love and affirmations, please do not hesitate to pass it to them.

My hope is that you will be blessed by this book, as will they be and that they can then also pay it forward and pass it on to another woman who may also benefit.

Thank you in advance and may God light your path!

About the Author

Dr. Christine Topjian is a multi-award winning author, educator, and wears many more hats each day. She loves to write books that show God's love and His provision for the world, helping each person tap into His best for their best lives.

Notes Section